FIRST WORD

Nowadays Alzheimer's Di[...] [...] in the media. Ten years ago [...] even by health professionals [...] ntia'. Now it is seen as an illne[...] h can begin at any age over about 40, [...] to old age. And with a rapidly increasing old [...] ain and other Western countries there is going to be [...] in the numbers of those with the illness and also those who look after them.

With 'Care in the Community' policies bringing changes to the world of care staff of all sorts, people are sometimes suddenly being faced with clients suffering from Alzheimer's Disease and other dementias, and may find that their behaviour is both puzzling and challenging. Hopefully 'Working with Alzheimer's Disease' will answer at least some of the questions and make it easier for staff to cope day by day; it may also help to ensure that people with Alzheimer's Disease are looked after with dignity and love at a time in their lives when everything seems to be falling apart.

My thanks are due to Sue Mitchell of Milton Court Resource Centre, Eastbourne, for reading the first draft, and to my wife, Chris, who read the proofs.

To James Hammond for the line drawings (which were in the original booklet editions)

To my son, Peter, a Fine Art Illustration student at Middlesex University for the design of the front cover and the drawing on page 56.

SECTION

ISBN 0 9514616 5 6

Working with Alzheimer's Disease
Fourth Edition (revised)

'Working with Alzheimer's Disease'

ISBN 0 9514616 5 6

1st Published 1988
4th Edition Revised 1994
1st Paperback Edition 1994

ULLSWATER PUBLICATIONS

SECTION A

WORKING WITH ALZHEIMER'S DISEASE

MAIN FEATURES

Alzheimer's disease is an illness which creeps up on a family quietly, without anyone really noticing that there is anything the matter. It's only afterwards that people begin to recall unusual events or behaviour patterns which were seen as 'one of those things', but with the benefit of hindsight were clearly important signs of trouble. It may seem as if a beloved older member of the family has changed in personality and started doing extraordinary things, but it's only much later that all the clues are put together and seen as part of an illness.

Usually people highlight particular behaviour problems. "My husband wanders off and gets lost'; "My wife doesn't know how to wash up any more. "My mother wets the bed every night'. But these are only symptoms of what is basically wrong with the Alzheimer brain: for those who work with Alzheimer's Disease it's important to find out what the underlying feature really is. Otherwise clients and their families will be treated wrongly and maybe unkindly just because staff have not understood what is likely to be happening in the damaged brains of the people they work with. For example, it's no use shouting at someone that you've already given them the cup of tea they asked for when they have no memory that they drank it ten minutes ago; it's no use claiming that an old lady is just being difficult or seeking attention when she won't get dressed in the morning and it's no use getting angry if you're accused of stealing her precious jewels or photos or money when she's hidden them at the back of a drawer.

So we need to start with a look at the most important features of Alzheimer's Disease and other dementias before dealing in detail with the various signs and symptoms which make life difficult and sometimes unbearable for families.

1. MEMORY LOSS

It seemed ridiculous that Frank couldn't remember the name of the town he lived in, and had no idea what he had done the day before especially when he had been off to see his latest grandchild. It seemed even more ridiculous that he could manage quite well to retell over and over again what happened when he was in the army in the second World War fighting in the North African desert. He seemed to have a clear memory of the home he was brought up in and also the one he moved into with his young bride in 1947. But to his wife's distress he often didn't seem to recognise her any longer and couldn't remember her name now. In fact, he seemed to think she was someone else and refused pointblank to go to bed with her or even share a room with her any longer.

Frank's memory loss may seem to be unusual, but it is typical of the problems of those who suffer from dementia. The recent past disappears from the mind within minutes even seconds; but there is still a clear and vivid recall of events long ago; or at least certain key events like getting married, a first job, a serious illness or an important event in the nation's life like the war or the coronation of the Queen.

I liken the memory to a video-tape. We are constantly recording new memories; at the same time we erase some of them either because they don't matter very much or because they are too painful for us. Unlike a video however, we can recall names, events, etc from many parts of the memory; looked at like this it's now more like a computer. But with someone suffering from Alzheimer's Disease the computer isn't always able to access the name or the event and the video tape has been erased in an unusual way – most things are erased immediately after they are recorded instead of being erased after some time. So it's not surprising that Frank can't remember the things that happened yesterday or maybe even five minutes ago. But not only are new events being erased, so are the old ones beginning with the most recent and going back ten, twenty, forty, even sixty years. And for some sufferers it is just as if they were living at that point in time. No wonder that Frank doesn't recognise his wife any longer, if he sees himself as a 25 year old; it might explain why he keeps on about going back home when he's lived in the same house for twenty years. Soon maybe he will have forgotten about his early married life and be looking for his mother and his childhood home or think that the Care Attendant is his school teacher.

This is known as short-term memory loss. It is the fundamental symptom of the illness. It may start with a loss of words, an inability to remember names of people and the names of things like everyday words such as 'table', 'door', 'cup', 'bus'.

So it affects conversation as important words disappear and the sentence remains unfinished; or maybe an alternative word is found to replace the one that has been forgotten; or the other person has to guess the word that is missing. It sets up a pattern of repeated stories from the part of the memory bank which remains intact like events in the war or a holiday long ago.

It affects relationships too. Frank's wife feels that he is deliberately trying to annoy her when he goes shopping and comes back with hardly anything. She's not very impressed with either excuses or reasons like ' You never told me to get the bread ', she just thinks he's being selfish. And when he forgets her birthday she begins to wonder if he loves her any longer; surely he isn't trying to organise a divorce at this stage in their married life!

At this point our own fears may begin to surface. Are our own lapses of memory a sign that Alzheimer's Disease has struck us too? The answer is probably not, especially before retirement age, where the percentage of people suffering from the illness is very small indeed. But it's true that all of us forget things. That is because they were not important enough for us to have entered them on the memory bank in the first place or because we had little use for them and discarded them along with all the other unimportant memories (like what we had for lunch three weeks ago last Friday). And then the final sign of a healthy memory; our ability to recall things, names, events, especially when we have stopped trying too hard. For example we may go up to our bedroom to get something, but be completely unable to remember what it was until we get downstairs again, when it suddenly comes back to us.

2. LOSS OF SKILLS

Memory doesn't stop with words and events and stories. Nearly all our skills have been learnt and put into our memory bank. And this is true whether we see ourselves as untrained and unskilled or whether we are highly trained in something special like Physics or Computing. All the ordinary things of life are skills that we learned once upon a time, even if we feel that they are automatic and we can do them without thinking. When we were born we were unable to dress ourselves or feed ourselves: these were skills which we had to master at an early age before we ever started on 'school' skills such as reading or writing. And there are many other examples, such as being toilet trained, tying shoelaces, brushing our hair, riding a bicycle which we take for granted and have no memory of ever having learnt.

With Alzheimer's Disease everything that has been learned can be unlearned: one skill can disappear from the active part of a person's skill-memory, whilst other skills are still active and unaffected. For example Mary stopped sending the weekly returns to Head Office because she couldn't remember how to fill in the details. It had been her job for five years and it wasn't really complicated; but now she had no idea of what she should do; she made up excuses, told lies, used her position as Head of the Department to keep other people quiet, until at last Head Office ran out of patience and the Managing Director demanded an explanation. They gave her early retirement on health grounds,but it was some time before the family realised that it wasn't stress and overwork that had been to blame.

Some skills demand a sequence of activities if they are to be done properly. For example researchers reckon that it takes 26 separate skills just to make a cup of tea, with sugar. Some sufferers get stuck in the middle of the activity. This time their brain is more like a broken record than a video-tape. They just repeat the latest little part of the sequence, just like the repeated line of a song, or a pianist who can't get away from the same bar of music. So, when Freda put her seventh teabag in the cup she was just repeating part of the sequence yet again without ever being able to get through to the end. It just needed someone to help her to move on to the next part of the sequence, and she would have managed perfectly. But all she succeeded in doing was making a cup of tea that nobody could drink.

A great many of our skills involve following a sequence of actions in the correct order and stopping at the end, not in the middle. Is this why Margaret tries to wear five skirts? She seems to carry on putting on skirts until she can't find any more to wear and doesn't seem to notice that she's getting hotter and hotter. Is this why John's sex life has fallen to pieces as he forgets how to make love and just falls off to sleep: not surprisingly his wife finds his advances now quite unacceptable. Is this why Ruth can't sit down? She may be stiff with arthritis but it's the damage to her brain which makes her refuse to sit in a chair sometimes: it's not that she doesn't want to sit down, it's simply that she can't remember the various skills involved in getting herself safely on to the chair.

Of course some days will be better than others. Freda may have no trouble in making the tea sometimes and Margaret may dress herself without any difficulty especially when there are visitors around and it's necessary to make a special effort. This is specially the case when there's a visit from the DSS doctor or when family members travel hundreds of miles to make their annual visit. It may appear that there is nothing wrong at all but neither Freda nor Margaret can be relied upon to make the tea or get dressed properly without supervision and help, even if they can manage to do well on special occasions.

3. LOSS OF SPATIAL AWARENESS

Why do people with Alzheimer's Disease fall over? For some it's a question of physical weakness as the disease gets to the stage where the body begins to waste away. Others may have forgotten the correct start to the sequence of moves for going down the stairs or pushing away from the kerb on a bicycle. In the confusion they end up on the floor or spreadeagled on the pavement.

But for others there may be an inability to know exactly where their hands and feet are: this may explain clumsy behaviour like missing the table and dropping the teacup plus its contents onto the floor. It may explain also why some people experience great difficulties with dressing and undressing (though there are other problems as well like an inability to recognise the clothes and remember the right sequence for putting them on).

Falls are also linked with the form of dementia called multi-infarct – a series of mini-strokes which are so insignificant as to go sometimes unnoticed. However some of them cause a momentary loss of consciousness which may well result in a person falling over; it might also be the cause of mystery accidents where car or train drivers have apparently made no attempt to slow down or stop before a head-on crash.

Writing skills can also be affected. As with people who have had a stroke, dementia sufferers may use only half the paper, leaving a huge margin, which they presumably are unaware of. Handwriting may become illegible, and there may be an inability to copy diagrams accurately.

4. FEELINGS

Alzheimer sufferers experience a range of feelings just as everyone else does. They are, however, often difficult to understand as the damaged brain sees the world and other people's actions in a way which makes very little sense to everyone else. But if your memory lasted only a few minutes, you would be likely to experience some of the extreme feelings which lead to unusual behaviour.

A few examples: if you had no idea where you were, you might be very frightened at being expected to walk into a place like a department store; if you couldn't remember names and faces you might well be frightened by a large family gathering; if you couldn't do a simple task like tying your shoelaces because you had forgotten how to do the job, you would find it frustrating, annoying and embarrassing. It could lead to feelings of depression, or else you might start blaming your nearest and dearest in an aggressive way.

If you couldn't find the words to express how you felt, you might well feel more and more isolated, imprisoned by a mind which no longer worked properly and in a world which was daily becoming more and more puzzling.

If you realised that you were no longer functioning properly and that things were getting worse, you might react with feelings of helplessness and despair.

Some of these feelings will be most apparent during the early stages of the illness, disappearing gradually as sufferers enter a period of their lives where they give the impression (in some cases) of being quite happy with their lives and unaware of the many problems that they cause their carers.

Alzheimer's Disease seems to attack the area of the brain which controls the emotions. There will be times when people laugh at things that would have offended them previously; similarly they may cry easily over things which really may be making them quite happy; so, if Grandma breaks down in floods of tears over the family photograph album, it may not be because she is distressed by the pictures from the past; she may be delighted, but is producing the wrong emotional response. (Of course, she may be really unhappy about it and the tears may reflect accurately the emotions of the moment).

Expressing love and anger may prove a problem as well. The old lady who wants to kiss everybody in the Day Centre every quarter of an hour can be difficult for some of the other regulars. So can the lady who appears naked in the hallway to greet visitors; or the man who thinks he's Don Juan and tries to make a pass at all the ladies in the Rest Home.

Anger may be the way that people can show their independence again. And for those in the final stages of the disease it may be one of the few means of communication left to them, as they find themselves moved about, toiletted, washed and dressed and fed as if they were infants. This may be necessary, but the powerlessness may well be resented, and needs to be acknowledged by those who do the caring. Anger may be very much reduced when clients are allowed to keep their dignity and are treated as adults even when the tasks that have to be done are similar to those that are done for a baby or very small child.

Carers' feelings can be seen as a mirror-image of some of the feelings of the person they are looking after. They may be angry at the way their lives have been disrupted; they may feel guilty that they are able to get out and about occasionally; they may experience fear that they will go out for half an hour and find their relative on the floor after a fall; they are likely to feel isolated and lonely because nobody calls any longer. This area of carers' feelings is dealt with in greater detail in section D.

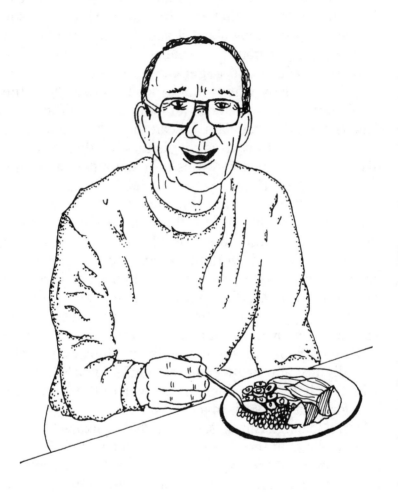

SECTION B

SYMPTOMS

1. WANDERING

The person with Alzheimer's disease who is found by the police standing outside the supermarket at three in the morning may seem to have wandered off. In practice it is likely that there is a purpose behind the wandering, but the patient had made a mistake which results from his loss of short-term memory.

a) He may have no idea what the time is.

b) He may just be unable to find the way home.

c) He may be trying to go to work.

d) He may be looking for his home, his school, his parents.

e) He may just want a breath of fresh air, or a short walk, or to do some window-shopping.

But unfortunately the outing goes wrong. He finds himself in an unknown street, perhaps only round the corner from where he came from, and is quite unable to find the way back. Those who are looking for a long-lost home may not realise that they are hundreds of miles away in another part of the country altogether; or they may be looking for a childhood home which has been demolished as a result of redevelopment (or even wartime bombing). And the people they are looking for will quite probably have moved away or be long since dead.

The wandering can therefore often be understood, but it still remains a major problem for the carer who may have to spend a lot of time and nervous energy combing the streets for a lost relative. Basic road sense can be affected by the illness, with some sufferers being picked up by the police, walking down the middle of the main road. The wanderer will probably be found by the police and eventually returned home, or a concerted effort by family and friends may be successful. Sometimes the wanderer may be very distressed at the realisation that he is lost and ordinary members of the public may find themselves with the problem on their hands. It would help them (and the police) if he or she were to wear an identity bracelet with name and address engraved on it.

Wandering often takes place in the middle of the night when the rest of the household is trying to sleep. It can be very worrying to hear footsteps on the stairs and down in the kitchen, and it may be necessary to get up and find out what is happening – just in case the house is about to be set on fire. Many sufferers from Alzheimer's disease seem to manage very well on a small amount of sleep (whilst the carer becomes more and more tired with caring on top of running a household and maybe holding down a job). And for some people with the illness there is no longer any idea of time, or of day and night. So, going out at night to do the shopping may be no more unreasonable than doing the same thing at 8 in the morning or at lunch-time. So, how can wandering be controlled? The carer may feel that there is no alternative to locking the doors and keeping the keys well and truly hidden. That may in practice be the only way of getting any peace and quiet: and it may also be the only way of making the quick trip round the corner to get a few items of shopping.

Policy among professionals seems to vary from place to place.

'Our front door is always open, at least during the daytime'. That may be the policy of a Residential Home which is prepared to run the risk that their residents may get well and truly lost. They will probably be trying to run the Home as 'normally' as possible and will feel that they have no right to curb the freedom of those who live there. After all they have not been deprived of their freedom by any court or any legal order.

'We make use of a second handle towards the top of the door'. Most people with dementia in homes where this is the policy have no idea how to operate the second handle as well as the usual one. It makes sure that residents only go out with the knowledge of staff.

'Our doors have an electronic device; it opens up if you know the combination number'. A very effective device for keeping people with dementia from getting out and perhaps being run over by the cars on the main road. And visitors can be given the number so that they don't have to find someone to let them out.

'We use a lock and key system. We have a responsibility to make sure that our clients don't put themselves at risk.' There are dangers in town in busy streets, but getting lost in the countryside may be even more dangerous as the wanderer may fall into water-filled ditches or die of exposure before they can be found.

'A small number of our residents wander off and are at considerable risk in the streets; so we use a tagging system which sets off an alarm as they pass through the front door.'

A variety of attitudes which reflect the expectations and philosophy of relatives and staff. They range from:

The relative; I chose that Home for my Dad because I wanted to make sure that he was safe all the time. I don't want them to let him get out onto that busy road; he'd probably walk in front of the traffic and get run over.

The manager: I want my home to be as normal as possible; so I don't intend to lock the clients up; most of them manage to find their way home again without any great difficulty. I feel that it's worth the risk.

The lawyer: You can't restrain people without going through the correct procedures. So you've got to use the relevant section of the Mental Health Act; and that means getting the doctor and the specialist Social Worker to come and make an assessment.

The neighbour: Sometimes an old lady comes and knocks on our front door; she seems to think that she lives here but in fact she lives in the Home round the corner. I just take her back there; it's no real trouble.

Another neighbour: These people at the Day Centre can be a big nuisance when they get lost in the streets. I think that the staff should make sure that they can't get out on their own.

There may, however, be ways of managing the problem without locks and bolts.

Night time wandering may be discouraged by daytime activities. For instance it may be a good idea for residents in a Home to be taken for a walk, maybe to the shops or out into the countryside if that is possible. Perhaps a bedtime drink may be helpful though this might cause an early morning trip to the toilet.

Daytime wanderers may need to be accompanied outside; but some may be perfectly capable of going a short distance on their own and it may be far better to risk someone getting lost than to create an atmosphere where the inmates are frustrated and angry.

There is also the whole question of the rights of the individual. Earlier in this century it seems that it was all too easy for some people to be placed in an institution and sometimes it was for very questionable reasons. Nowadays the law requires a Doctor and a designated Social Worker to use their powers under the Mental

Health Act to remove someone to a secure unit for their own safety or the safety of others. Quite reasonably these are powers which are made use of only on rare occasions; freedom is not something to be thrown away lightly. So it's not perhaps right for a Care Home owner to agree with neighbours who think that 'the old lady shouldn't be allowed to wander off like that'. Perhaps they should just be prepared to help guide her back home from time to time.

2. THE AGGRESSIVE SUFFERER

Some people have been aggressive all their lives; Alzheimer's Disease may make them worse. Others have been placid and easy going all their lives; Alzheimer's Disease may make them appear to have changed completely in personality as they develop an aggressive approach to others both in word and action.

The explanation may be obvious in some cases. They may be like Edith who found herself in a Residential Home but had no idea where she was or who all the strangers were who helped to get her washed and dressed and organised her life for her. What she wanted was to get back to the home she loved. She couldn't understand that that was no longer possible as there was no way that she could look after herself any more. Edith couldn't remember where her room was; she had no idea where to find the toilet and spent the day in a constant state of anxiety. She was also confused and angry when she was made to get up and go into the dining room for a meal that she didn't want to eat. It shouldn't have been surprising that she started to be aggressive to everyone in sight, both residents and staff.

Anger may also be the result of a carer's actions or words. Charles was quite happy wearing his hat in bed; he was doing no harm to anyone. But his wife felt embarrassed and told him in no uncertain terms to take it off. When he took no notice she snatched it from him and hid it under the bed. Charles' fury was something his wife had never witnessed before. and he only calmed down when she gave way and he was able to wear his hat again.

Behaviour like this is known as a catastrophic reaction. To the person with Alzheimer's Disease the carer's actions may seem totally unreasonable and unloving and he responds in a way which is more like the reaction of a small child to the removal of a favourite toy.

So, what's the answer? Simply to avoid a confrontation if at all possible; and many situations do not need to be treated confrontationally. Charles' hat was eccentric but not dangerous; so he could have been left to wear it. And there are lots of similar examples. Does it really matter if someone eats their meal with a spoon instead of a knife and fork? Is it worth a major row to insist that the apples must definitely go in the fruit bowl and not in the kitchen cupboard?

This doesn't mean that carers have to accept everything that their relative demands. Setting light to the furniture is something that must be stopped immediately. But most other behaviour problems are annoying or embarrassing rather than dangerous; gentle persuasion or diversion to some other activity might be much more effective than risking an explosion of anger which is likely to leave everybody exhausted.

Some aggressive behaviour seems to have no obvious cause, just a surge of energy which takes everyone by surprise, specially when the person is normally unable to do a great deal for himself.

3. THE PASSIVE SUFFERER

Ruth never said much; she sat in her chair in the corner and did nothing most of the day. She never complained or made a fuss; the staff saw her as a 'good' client, unlike all the others who made a noise or shouted or flew into a temper at the slightest thing. But Ruth's passive behaviour really had the same cause. She too was powerless; she too did not know where she was and longed for a home which she could never return to. But instead of being aggressive she seemed to accept everything and allowed the world to pass her by. She showed some of the signs of depression; but that's not surprising in the circumstances. I might be depressed if I realised that I was losing memory and skills but still retained a vague understanding that this was not my home.

A passive pattern of behaviour poses fewer problems to the carer and maybe is seen as ideal as it enables the work of the house (or Home or the ward) to be done much more easily. It should not, however be seen as desirable just because it leads to an easier life. Passive sufferers need to be stimulated with a range of activities (See section C. How to manage the person with Alzheimer's Disease page 33).

4. REPEATED QUESTIONS

When Uncle Eric rang up for the fourth time to ask which train he should catch for his visit, his niece began to realise for the first time that something was wrong with his memory. Up till then Uncle had always been so efficient. He had always been keen on travelling and had always made his own arrangements; but this time he seemed quite unable to remember that it was the 11 o/clock train that they had decided on. Eventually she wrote it down and sent it off in the post.

Uncle Eric knew that he was developing a memory problem and was very apologetic about being a nuisance. But others whose dementia has developed into the middle stage of the illness carry on asking the same question over and over again. It may seem to be a deliberate attempt to be annoying, but in reality the patient has completely forgotten what the answer to the question was. He may want to know when lunch is going to be ready, but even at the fifth or sixth time of asking he has no idea what the answer is, and has even forgotten that he has asked the question already. He may have just come back from a drive in the country, but have no idea whether it is still something to look forward to, or whether it's an activity which is over. Imagine how distressing it must be for the patient to be answered in an angry tone of voice when all he did was to ask for a cup of tea, or what the time is. He doesn't know that he's been asking the same question for the past ten minutes, and so comes to the conclusion that those who look after him are being quite unfair and unkind to him. On the other hand the carer may have got to the point of desperation and in a moment of anger says things which are unkind and hurtful which may be immediately regretted.

The answer to the problem for both carer and the care assistant is to try to divert the sufferer's attention to another activity, so that within a couple of minutes he has completely forgotten all about the questions which were in his mind. For those who can still read with understanding it will be helpful if basic activities of the day can be written down; the carer can refer to the list and point out to the sufferer where he has got to in the day's programme. We all need a calendar and diaries to help jog our own memory, so a more extensive diary or series of lists can be helpful to a person whose brain is damaged. However, it's easy to imagine that a person is able to understand when in practice they have no idea of the meaning of the words they are reading.

5. INAPPROPRIATE BEHAVIOUR

Little children sometimes attract attention by taking their clothes off at unsuitable moments; so can people with Alzheimer's disease. But it's much more of a shock to find Granny removing her bra and knickers in the living room than it is when a 2 year old does a similar strip-tease.

Of course Granny may just be too hot, and the part of her brain which deals with tact and correct social behaviour has been damaged. As a result it may seem quite normal to walk down the road half naked on a summer's day, or bring the fire nearer to her on a cold day by piling the burning coal in the middle of the carpet.

Ordinary tact may also disappear and a person may say exactly what he is thinking – to the embarrassment of all around. For instance he might make an unflattering comment on a lady's new hairstyle or recently bought dress; he might ask probing questions about a stranger's life style; he might go in for risqué jokes which are out of character. There might be no problems in public until all of a sudden, when the carer's guard is down, something occurs which threatens to create a dispute in public. When John's father came to stay, he took him off down to the Lamb for a pint or two; it was crowded and they had to share a small table with other people who were having a lunchtime sandwich garnished with tomato. Suddenly Dad reached across and took the lady's tomato from her plate. John could feel himself going red with embarrassment as the lady stared in surprise at what had just happened. Fortunately John's knowing wink won the day; no comments were made; no questions were asked. But John knew that he would have to be much more careful when he took his Dad down to the pub on other occasions – other people might be less easily dealt with next time.

Shopping can be a minefield. For some people with Alzheimer's Disease there is a sort of hoarding instinct which can result in the cupboard being stacked out with vast quantities of goods which are never used. Worse still is the problem regarding the loss of the sense of what is legal. Just as it's necessary for parents to keep a watch on their small children as they pass through the supermarket check-out, so does the carer need to keep an eye on their dementing relative, who may be just as likely to pocket a bar of chocolate from the display near the exit. The difference is that the shopkeeper may be far less sympathetic and might insist on calling the police and pressing shoplifting charges. It may be worthwhile to warn the local shop-keepers about the problem in advance of any actual difficulty, but bigger stores or ones in a holiday town may prove to be a bigger problem.

Unusual behaviour may also be caused by fear of the unknown or the totally new. Grandad may refuse to get on to a new type of bus because it has a different sort of entrance which he finds frightening; as a result he makes a scene in public which may give the carer a first taste of embarrassing problems. The answer is not to withdraw from contact with others, but instead to try to explain briefly and frankly the problem of looking after a brain-damaged person (without of course embarrassing the sufferer).

6. SPEECH PROBLEMS

Mary tells long stories which make no sense to anyone else; it's more like listening to one long riddle.

Arthur starts a sentence, but stops when he gets half way through. He usually stops after the word 'the' or 'a'; he's completely forgotten the name of the thing or the person, and just tails off.

Fred has got to the stage of the illness where he can't do much more than say a few words. The rest of the time he's wrapped up in his own thoughts.

In all three cases conversation becomes very difficult: so there's a temptation for care assistants and nurses to ignore the sufferer and talk to each other across the bed or chair while they get on with the work of caring for the sufferer's bodily needs. The sufferer at home may also feel isolated if there are a lot of people talking; it may be impossible to follow what is being said, and very easy to say something ridiculous. Equally the carer who looks after a sufferer on his/her own may be condemned to a world of silence, as meaningful conversation dies out. It is easy to assume that people who do not talk can't understand what is being said over them and around them. But we know that some people who are apparently unconscious are able to recall vividly conversations which were not meant for their ears. Similarly people who have had a stroke may be able to understand everything, but have no way of making any reply which can be understood by others. So it is quite likely that people with Alzheimer's Disease may be able to understand even if there is no obvious sign that they are doing so.

But feelings continue even when words have lost their meaning. So, the way in which people are spoken to, will reflect the love and care of a Home or a carer; or alternatively it can reflect neglect and lack of concern.

I feel therefore that staff and relatives should be extremely careful not only about their words, but also about the tone of voice and body language that they use. They need to avoid talking to other staff while doing a job like dressing or washing someone, but instead, to talk to the person that they are caring for; otherwise they will give the impression that they are just dealing with a body, rather than with a person with a history, a personality and feelings.

There may be special problems for people whose mother tongue is not English. They have spent the first part of their life in a country like Bangladesh or India and came to Britain as immigrants thirty years ago; others may have come from a European country and stayed here after getting married. As English may have been learned as an adult, it is quite possible for that skill to disappear, leaving the mother tongue as the only available language. The effects of this will vary from person to person. For some who live within their own community without much contact with English speakers it may not cause many problems. However, there will be others who are isolated from their homeland and culture; for them there may be a complete breakdown of communication with neighbours and with family. They may have children who have never learnt the language and grandchildren who may never even have visited the country that they came from or have the slightest interest in doing so. For people in this position it seems essential that an effort is made to find volunteers who can speak the language and ideally be from the same community.

7. DIFFICULTIES WITH DRESSING

Dressing correctly is a complicated exercise, which we take several years to learn properly until it becomes automatic. But Alzheimer's Disease involves a loss of skills which may make clothes as much of a puzzle to a sufferer as if he was a 2 year old; neither can identify the clothes properly; so trousers may become the latest sort of headgear; button and buttonholes can easily be mismatched and make the person look like a clown.

The Alzheimer patient has two even bigger problems. Most children are learning all the time, but Alzheimer's Disease leads gradually to the loss of one skill after another. Furthermore the sufferer may not know where the various parts of the body are. Imagine not being able to locate where your feet are! This combined with a lack of understanding of the meaning of nouns may make dressing a matter of pure guesswork, and a cause of great frustration for those who are trying to help.

Just as children can be obstructive and unco-operative about the clothes they wear, so can the Alzheimer's Disease patient. He may refuse to get into pyjamas to go to bed, or insist on going around the house in a dressing-gown for most of the day. If persuasion won't alter things, it may be necessary to accept this sort of behaviour. It may be unusual, but it's not really necessary to make a big issue out of it; there will probably be more important things to worry about.

8. INCONTINENCE

A child will have probably mastered the complex skill of being dry and clean by the age of two or three. Accidents may happen in the next few years, but it can be a big embarrassment for a family to find the accidents happening in middle or old age and to a respected senior member of the family.

It can, however, be a temporary problem which can happen to anyone as a result of an infection or an illness, but for the Alzheimer patient it's yet another failure in the downhill progress of the illness, and also one which has terrible social consequences – excursions out of the house become much more difficult to organise, above all on public transport, and visitors are understandably put off from coming to the house. So incontinence spells isolation.

There are several causes:

1. Not knowing the bladder or bowels need to be emptied, because the brain no longer sends the correct signals to this area of the body.
2. Not knowing where the toilet is. In some cases all the doors to the rooms of the house look the same, and there is no memory of what lies behind them. For other people the toilet is no longer where they expect it to be; i.e. in childhood it may have been outside or even at the bottom of the garden, but it's no longer there and the sufferer can't find it.
3. Mistaking one receptacle for another; the waste paper basket may just appear to be the same shape to the sufferer.
4. Not being able to move fast enough to get to the toilet in time (this applies to other elderly people as well).

Suggestions to meet the problem are dealt with in Section C9 page 48.

9. DANGEROUS BEHAVIOUR

Ted had been a smoker all his life and used matches to light his pipe. One day he couldn't find his matches, so he tore off some of the daily paper, made a spill out of it, and lit it on the gas fire in the living room. When it flared up, he dropped it, and it set some other papers alight.

Ellen put the potatoes on to boil; she poured enough water into the pan, but after she had turned on the electricity, she just forgot what she was doing, and went back to the living room. Eventually she smelt burning, but didn't link it with any action of hers. So she left it to burn away.

Most of the stories like these are a problem for carers in the home, who haven't got the time for proper supervision, particularly if they have to be out of the house for long periods of time (to go to work for example) and it's also a major worry for Social Workers and others when they are responsible for a dementing person who lives alone.

It may be necessary to take drastic steps to avoid accidents e.g. by turning off the gas supplies or going over to central heating.

However, for the care attendant working on a sitter service, cooking is a very suitable activity. In some ways it can be similar to the cooking a mother may do with a small child, where it's a co–operative venture with a lot of supervision.

Similarly there is no reason why the Residential Home and the Day Centre cannot do the same, provided that there is enough supervision. The results may be a great boost to a person's confidence, and the activity itself has value in providing stimulation.

Some families find themselves with the totally

unexpected. May was so weak that she could hardly get up out of a chair without help. But one day she became very agitated, rushed to the front door and was off and away before her sister had time to stop her; and worse still she went so fast down the hill that nobody managed to catch up with her before she got to the main road and dashed straight across without a glance towards the traffic. Fortunately there were no vehicles just at that moment, but it was an anxious few minutes before May was safely back home and calmed down again. Her sister needed some calming down as well.

There are also some people suffering from Alzheimer's who can get very angry particularly with those who are looking after them.

Gerald was afraid that his wife would pick up something like a knife or a fork and stab him; so he never turned his back on her just in case. It's unlikely that she would have managed to organise a proper attack but Gerald wasn't going to take the risk.

And there are also those who have got to the later stages of the illness where they may still have some strength but have lost all sense of the need for self-protection. In these situations carers can find themselves trapped inside their own home unable to get to the shop at the end of the road or even to the garage to fetch something. And they may have to rig up a device to wake them in the night to make sure that they don't find that their relative has fallen down the stairs and is lying in a crumpled heap at the bottom. For them the work of the Care Attendant is specially valuable: otherwise their care easily becomes a 24 hour round-the-clock affair.

10. TEARS – LAUGHTER

When the family visited Maurice, he regularly burst into tears at some stage in the afternoon; they all found this very upsetting and thought that he must be dreadfully unhappy. It seemed to be linked with music and photographs; so they stopped bringing the photos in to the Home. That just made the visit a little more difficult. But Maurice's emotional control was damaged, and he was no longer able to find the appropriate response. In fact both the music and the photos were giving him a lot of pleasure (though of course some gave him sad memories as well), but he wasn't able to express his pleasure in the way he used to be able to. We sometimes say we don't know whether to laugh or cry. Maurice was even more unsure, and the memories that gave him pleasure also brought tears to his eyes and embarrassment to the family.

Laughter is similar. Alzheimer sufferers may find things riotously funny, when previously they would not have been amused at all. In fact they might have been very offended. They can also laugh at the wrong moment, just as children can do. They have lost the inhibitions which keep most of us from laughing too obviously when someone slips on a banana skin. There are times when such an ability to laugh is an acute embarrassment, but it can also relieve tension, above all if everyone is able to share the joke. Alzheimer's Disease can be a depressing illness for all concerned. So the moments when we can laugh with people can be very precious and a means of healing the wounds and hurts which can be the experience of the Alzheimer sufferer. It is, however, important to underline how hurtful it is for the sufferer if anyone laughs at him/her because of silly mistakes or odd behaviour. It is vital that they are respected as people of value and dignity and never as objects of fun.

11. MONEY – VALUABLES

"Sandra's taken my purse. It had £10 in it and it's gone." Sandra had been Mum's Home Help for three years, and there was no doubt about it: Sandra could be relied on 100%; there was no way that she could have taken Mum's purse. Of course it was eventually found down the side of the front room settee, where Mum had put it for safe keeping. But unfortunately she had forgotten all about it and assumed it had been stolen. Fortunately she didn't accuse Sandra to her face or call the police, but she might have done.

A month later it was grandson John in the firing line. He'd done Mum's shopping for her – a loaf of bread, some jam and the local newspaper. Total cost £1.26. There was 24p change which he'd handed over straightaway, but five minutes after he'd got home Mum was on the phone saying he'd kept the change. She'd forgotten about the three coins on the mantelpiece.

Next it was her jewellery that was missing. Sandra arrived for work to find a police car outside the door and a young policeman busily writing the details of the crime in his notebook. Sandra said she thought she knew where they might be, and, sure enough, there they were in the cupboard in the spare bedroom, the favourite hiding–place of the previous few weeks. The policeman closed up his notebook with a sigh. At the front door Sandra had a quick word to try to explain the situation – Mum wasn't really trying to waste his time, she just regularly forgot where she put things; and then she just assumed that they had been stolen; after all it was much less threatening to her than having to admit that she was losing her memory.

Alzheimer's Disease destroys the memory of the recent past. People like Mum would have no recollection of what happened to the purse or the change or the jewellery, even although she would probably have a very good memory for events and people further back in time. The most likely people to be accused of theft are Home Helps, Care Attendants, sitters, workmen and members of the family, many of whom may be working very hard to try to cope with the problems posed by someone suffering from Alzheimer's Disease.

It's important not to become upset by unfair accusations. Instead steps need to be taken to reduce the chances of a major dispute. Sandra had a good idea where to look for the jewellery; but it won't always be a place like a cupboard; it might be the waste paper basket or down the loo. On the other hand it would have been a good idea for John to have left a written note of what he had bought for his Gran and how much change he had brought back with him.

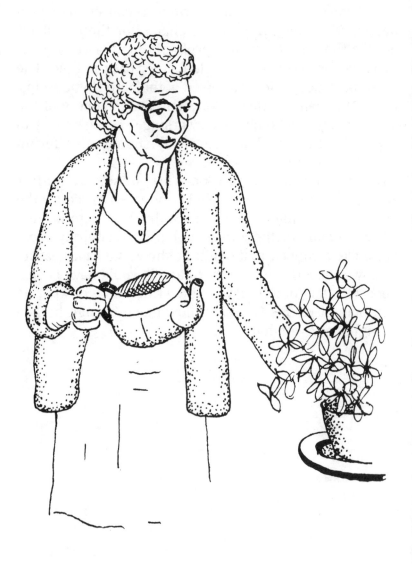

SECTION C

HOW TO MANAGE THE PERSON WITH ALZHEIMER'S DISEASE

1. REALITY ORIENTATION

Most of us have a huge range of common–sense knowledge. We picked it up long ago, perhaps when we were children; for example we recognise coins and banknotes; we know how to tell the time; we know which shop to go to when we want to buy a newspaper.

We use diaries, calendars, shopping lists to help us; we have dictionaries to help us spell; we use cookery books to remind us of a recipe we last used six months ago. We also recognise and name things which are important to us, the parts of a car, the special words used in our hobby, as well as ordinary words like the names for flowers and birds; but we may also need to look things up in a DIY book or get a friend to explain how to do a job or check out the name of something. And we use a variety of other methods to help us rather than remember every item of information that we might need. We use diaries, calendars and shopping lists; we don't remember every address and phone number that we need; instead we rely on the telephone directory and our address book.

The damaged Alzheimer brain needs help far more often as names disappear and skills vanish. One way of helping is through Reality Orientation (or RO for short). At its simplest that is an extension of the diaries and calendars that we all have. Some Homes and Day Centres have an RO board with simple information such as: date, day of the week, weather, the name of the Home, the name of the town, what meal is the next one. For those who can read and understand, it is very valuable to be able to go and check on certain basic questions for themselves. It saves staff time, it enables people to be less dependant on others for information, as they can check up on what they want to know as often as they want to.

There is however, a problem with the RO board: Out–of–date information.

One example:

It was Thursday afternoon when a group of us went to take the service at the Home, but according to the RO board it was Remembrance Sunday. Four days of confusion for residents if they bothered to take any notice. So it should be stressed that the RO board must be changed first thing in the morning every morning, and altered during the day where necessary. Otherwise in my opinion it should be scrapped as it is likely to do more harm than good.

The RO board is very limiting and should be seen as just one aspect of Reality Orientation. It can be used as a basis for group work where all the basic information is gathered from members of the group. This may take as much as half an hour to complete if the people taking part are very limited.

But more attractive from the point of view of the staff is the wide–ranging topic work which can be undertaken by people in the earlier stages of the illness. People may need to be reminded of some of the ordinary things of life in the 90s. For example decimal currency may be a mystery to someone who may only be able to think in terms of pounds shillings and pence as they were taught when they were at school. Another theme is current events – items from local and national newspapers might be of interest and give opportunities for discussion and maybe for people to show off their expertise.

However, Reality Orientation is not best seen as something which takes half an hour like any other activity in a well run Centre or Home. In fact RO should be a 24 hour a day policy in which every member of staff keeps each client informed of simple basic things through ordinary friendly conversations. This could include the weather, the time of year, the flowers in the garden, the photographs that are on the table. It is also important for members of staff to introduce themselves each time they are dealing with someone: it's quite likely that they will not be recognised as the same person who was on duty the day before and it will just seem that there is a constant stream of new and strange faces passing through the establishment. It may also be necessary to remind clients where they are living or which Day Centre they are attending. Even without the difficulties of a dementing illness it's always possible for people in Nursing Homes to lose touch with their surroundings and to exist in a sort of vacuum. With dementia it is to be expected that people lose track of where they are living and as a result try to wander off, looking for the home of earlier times; and it's also not surprising when they don't recognise friends, family and staff or muddle them with someone from their past. 24 hour RO may not answer all the problems, but it does help to minimise them.

2. REMINISCENCE THERAPY

As long–term memory is affected at a later stage, patients with Alzheimer's Disease may still have vivid memories of events of childhood or early married life or times of great change or danger like the World Wars. Getting them to talk about their experiences and knowledge gives them an opportunity to be experts again at a time when modern technology seems to be leaving them behind.

The following ideas may prove to be useful and stimulating both with individuals and in group work.

a Old tools, farming implements etc. can provide a talking point about working life in the past.

b) 'What did you do in the war?'

c) Articles from a time spent abroad, a spear from Africa for example.

d) Old photographs, either of the town or village as it used to be seventy years ago, or of members of the family.

e) Old songs, ranging from Music Hall and the Jazz era to hymns remembered from Sunday School (for younger sufferers classic hits might be the right sort of music).

f) A 'This is your Life' scrap–book, built up with the help of relatives and friends.

All this can lead to discussion not only between older and younger, but can provide opportunity for reminiscence among those who come to a Day Centre and can be a source of great pleasure to them; but there are other advantages too. Photographs from the past can be linked to present–day ones which will assist with the 24 hour RO which should be happening; and it doesn't have to be confined to pictures of the local pub and the village church. It can also involve pictures of everyday items past and present; cookers, cars, typewriters, clothing are just a few examples. All this may encourage conversation and stimulate people's memories; it gives opportunity for staff and family and friends to get alongside the person with Alzheimer's Disease and provide an activity which can be shared. And usually this is an activity which gives pleasure.

Tears may come, but this is not necessarily a sign of unhappiness or sorrow (though it may be). It may instead be the result of the damage to the part of the brain which deals with the emotions which doesn't always send out the right signals. As a result tears may come at the wrong moment.

One further benefit concerns the staff. Reminiscence gives an insight into the life story of a person. Freda is no longer 'the one who sits by the window'. She's a wife and mother, a grandmother too, she's a lady who has travelled the world and worked hard as a volunteer. Joe is a father and grandfather, somebody who once had responsibility for hundreds of workers; he stops being the person who spends his time pacing up and down the corridors. Maggie was the manageress of a local shop; her expertise as a dressmaker was the talk of the town. Now that she can't remember what to do with a needle and thread, she can get some pleasure from the pictures in her scrap–book and talk with the staff about times past, (though she may only be able to do the listening).

3. EXCURSIONS, WALKS

Carers may be afraid for the safety of relatives outside the home if there is any possibility that they will wander off or behave dangerously when crossing the road. That is particularly understandable when the carer is physically frail or has difficulty walking (or running!). But many people with Alzheimer's are fit and strong and will find it very frustrating to be kept indoors when they would like to be outside. This is specially the case in the earlier stages of the illness when it seems that there are no signs of an illness, just peculiar behaviour.

The management of residential homes should make sure that there is a programme which includes regular trips out. Shopping expeditions, a trip to a pub, a walk in the country, a visit to a service at the nearby church, a coach trip to the seaside – all these are possible activities.

Of course there are people with Alzheimer's who are frightened by being outside the security of the home; and there are others who are too frail to cope with such an expedition. But that is not an excuse for leaving people just to stare at a television screen.

The person who wants to go for a walk should be allowed to do so – safely. Good design of buildings and gardens will make it possible for people to walk on their own without getting into difficulties. For example paths designed in a figure–of–eight or a circle will make it easier for people to find their way back to the building without involving the staff. In other situations that will not be possible. So staff should expect to take people out from time to time perhaps to the park or to the shops or just a hundred yards down the street and back again. Shortage of staff may make this difficult at times, but management and budgets should allow for this sort of activity.

Sitters in the private home may feel that they would like to do the same: but they must make sure that they have the agreement of their supervisor and the relative.

Anyone taking a person with Alzheimer's out is taking a risk (one which I feel is worth taking). Here are some of the problems:

a) Getting the patient to come back again. Are you sure that you can rely on their co–operation above all when the time comes to go back home? Just in case there are difficulties it may be wise to select a circular route.

b) If you use a bus, are you sure that the problem of finding a seat (perhaps while you're paying the driver) won't lead to some panic reaction?

c) If you use your car, are you sure that your passenger won't suddenly grab the wheel and cause an accident?

d) Are you insured when you're out in the streets? Does your own car insurance cover you?

4. ACTIVITIES AT HOME / IN THE DAY CENTRE / IN THE RESIDENTIAL HOME.

Left to themselves, many people with Alzheimer's drop off into a world of their own or alternatively become a minor nuisance as they wander about aimlessly. But with a proper programme of activities they may be able to retain skills and regain some of the confidence which has been lost during the course of the illness.

This is perhaps most easily done at the Day Centre. Clients may come for a few hours or an entire working day, and most Centres see their role as one of providing a range of activities. The carer on his or her own may find activities extremely difficult to arrange. It may be all that the carer can do to keep the house clean and tidy and to see that their relative is washed, dressed, toiletted and fed. To expect to play games, read books, supervise cooking is more than they may be able to cope with, and it may therefore be the job of the Day Centre or a sitter to fill the gap.

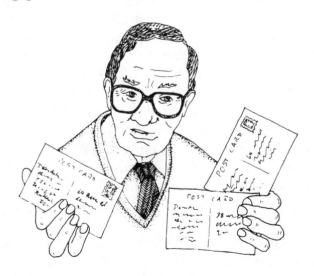

The residential home should be a place of activity; perhaps 'Rest Home' is a title that gives the wrong impression to staff and families alike. There should be a programme of activities which residents are encouraged to take part in and which should be the particular responsibility of a member of staff or a visiting organiser. Often, however, shortage of staff and shortage of vision can lead to residents being left in their rooms on their own or parked in a lounge with a flickering TV screen for company; in this sort of home the organiser of activities is at a real disadvantage; he/she may be seen as a nuisance, and the difficulty of getting residents ready for the activity gives a good excuse to return to a very basic pattern of care.

So, what can be done to provide the stimulation that is needed to encourage alertness?

Residential homes and Day Centres can develop programmes of individual and group activity, some of which may also be suitable for the sufferer in the home. Many things that are suitable for children will also appeal to the Alzheimer patient, unless of course, they are obviously childish. Many games are labelled 'age 6 to adult' and can involve the whole family; jigsaw puzzles can be good as long as they don't appear to be aimed at the pre-school child who appreciate Donald Duck pictures a little more than Grandad will. It's very important that the Alzheimer patient is not made to feel as if he's being treated as child. Games of skittles or quoits are also good, but many games which are suitable for younger people may require a speed of reaction which is beyond the ability of a brain-damaged person.

Some skills may be damaged beyond repair, but it is possible that with a little bit of help others will be restored at least to some extent. It will be helpful to discover what hobbies, skills and interests a person had before their illness. The following might be worthwhile, as long as the necessary facilities can be provided on the premises.

Carpentry, though it will require a lot of supervision. Pottery, painting, knitting, sewing, craftwork, cooking – perhaps with a lot of help. Gardening, both indoors and outdoors. Helping around the house. Some residents will be only too keen to dust or clean, perhaps doing the same job over and over again. They may also be able to set the table or clear away and wash up.

Some of these domestic activities require the co–operation and active support of domestic staff in the kitchen. Or, alternatively there should be a second kitchen available for residents to practise their skills, without getting in the way of the preparation of the meals for the whole establishment.

Go into the lounge of many a residential home and the television set will be playing: perhaps to a sleeping audience. So, what's the purpose of having it on? I suspect it helps to give staff a quiet life whilst providing an impression of activity. Unfortunately most people with Alzheimer's don't really understand what's going on, as TV moves too fast for their damaged brain. As a result it is unlikely to give the stimulation that it gives to other people. And, it may also be so confusing that it provides a form of Unreality Orientation, in which the real world and the fantasy world of the small screen get mixed up, providing good opportunities for increasing the delusions that can occur anyway.

For the carer in the home the TV may provide a welcome break from the constant demands of looking after someone single–handed. In the Day Centre and residential Home I feel that its use should be limited, so that everyone is encouraged to think in terms of activity.

5. MUSIC, DANCE, SINGING.

Alzheimer's disease leaves certain parts of the brain unaffected until the last stages of the illness. Speech may become difficult to understand; memory may be nearly non–existent, but musical skills and appreciation carry on relatively undamaged. What is more, there are some people who have been unable to speak at all, who have managed to sing the lines of a well–known song which they learned earlier in life.

This provides clue no 1 for successful management; find the right sort of music for the sufferer, and he or she may well be happy for hours. It may be light music or classical; it may be the songs of the 1920s or 1930s or even the popular tunes of the first World War or the Music Hall era. It is far more likely to provide stimulation than the TV and will give pleasure to carer and cared–for alike. It may lead to a sing–song in the living–room or a knees–up in the Day Centre. Both are good for general health and give an opportunity for valuable exercise. Both are community activities which will often be welcomed by older people who spend a lot of time on their own or just with one relative.

Suitable music is not difficult to find: records, tapes and radio will provide a wide range to meet the needs and tastes of people of all ages and backgrounds. The Winslow Press catalogue offers for example '30 Years of Popular Music', Max Bygraves', 'SingaLonga War Years' and a 'Sing Along Tape', selections from the Winslow Song Book (large–print). There's also a series of videos called 'Music, Memories and Milestones' which includes music from the 30s to the 60s as part of its contents. It includes the Rock'n'Roll years, the Beatles as well as the Big Bands and Gracie Fields.

Playing a musical instrument is a skill to be cherished: but it can easily be neglected if other family members don't share the same musical interest. Granny's piano may have had to be sold when she moved in to other accommodation, and other instruments may be packed away out of sight. So the visit to the Day Centre may give a good opportunity for people to practise their skills; or in the home the sitter who comes once a week might have musical skills which he/she can share with the client. The repertoire of music remembered from days long ago can be encouraged, but there are cases of people with dementia who are able to learn new pieces of music even although they may have great difficulty with other skills.

Hymn singing is another good community activity which can also be used in the home. Modern hymns and choruses are likely to be a problem with unfamiliar tunes and words which will probably be unhelpful and puzzling. As with other areas of life it's better to concentrate on the old favourites using books such as Hymns Ancient & Modern, Moody & Sankey, Golden Bells. The local church could be invited into the Day centre or residential Home to help with a service but all those taking part should be expected to undergo some simple form of training so that they have some idea of the needs of people with dementia.

Music may solve some problems. But it can also create others. Isobel was an opera singer when she was young. Now she can only remember the first few notes of the opera that made her famous. George used to be able to play a range of different pieces on the piano; now he can only remember one or two, and other people don't always appreciate hearing the same thing over and over again. Henry's memory musical memory goes round in circles; he gets to the end of a bar and starts again at the beginning of the piece so that he never manages to get to the end of it. As with other memory problems of this sort it may just need someone to nudge him on to the next bar and let him escape from a sort of vicious circle.

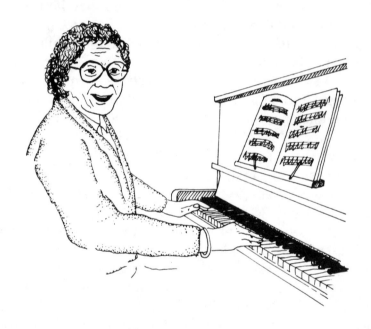

6. NON–CONFRONTATION

Arguing with someone with Alzheimer's Disease is only likely to make a difficult situation worse. Except in cases of really dangerous behaviour it's best to take a non-confrontational approach to problems.

As with small children success may come through diversion to some other activity. For example, it may be annoying to have someone pacing up and down the living room for long periods of time. Perhaps a walk in the garden or down the road might deal with the need for a breath of fresh air. Of course, they may need to be accompanied and brought safely back home.

Some behaviour may be just eccentric; using a spoon instead of a knife and fork may not be the normal way to eat a main meal, but it's unwise to insist on 'proper' behaviour, even if it causes the carer some embarrassment in public or when visitors come.

There's no need to tell someone off for bad behaviour. Picking up someone else's things is not the same as stealing, even if the owner is upset about the loss. People with Alzheimer's Disease don't have the same sense of ownership that they would have had earlier in life. What they need is to be gently told that the article belongs to someone else, and then find something which will divert their attention to something else.

And there's no need to get upset when someone goes to get their coat for the sixth time in ten minutes. It may be a bit frustrating to have to tell a client yet one more time that it's too early for the transport home, but he or she will have forgotten what you said within a very short time, and will still be anxious to be ready on time.

An angry or agitated response by a care worker is likely to wrongly interpreted by people with Alzheimer's. They will have no idea why you appear to be angry and are shouting at them. They will just thing that it's *you* who is unreasonable and that you don't love them any more.

Equally there's no future in using logic. It may be annoying to find the dining-room floor nearly covered in sugar, but it won't help to waste time on explaining that that's the wrong way to help to prepare for the next meal. It's best to gently divert the person to another job such as putting out the cutlery or getting something from the kitchen. That will give time to clear up the mess without fuss and bother.

Of course, where behaviour is dangerous there is no time for arguing or diverting. It may be necessary to take a knife off someone, or hide the matches, or just get out of the way for the moment.

7. ENCOURAGEMENT

'Silly old granny', says Michael, as the old lady tries to eat her soup with a knife. He may well be copying his parents who have had many a trying month since Granny came to stay. Nonetheless, despite the problems Granny does not need to have her inadequacies and difficulties highlighted by anyone, least of all her 5 year old grandson. (It won't do him much good either!) But Granny's happiness will not be increased by the family's attitude. She needs to be told how well she is doing when she succeeds in dressing herself properly, or doing a simple piece of knitting. She needs to be shown how much they love her and respect her, even when she makes mistakes or has some sort of accident.

The same applies to all who help in any way, in home, hospital or Day Centre. That may mean that you avoid using terms like 'luv' or 'grandad' unless you know for certain that that is what a person wishes to be called. It may also mean talking to the person instead of across them to the other member of staff who is working with you on a job like changing a bed or cleaning up after someone has been incontinent. It also means trying to avoid making sufferers unnecessarily dependent on the staff, with the result that they are treated as if they were small children.

8. BODY, MIND, SPIRIT

Alzheimer patients need to be stimulated; otherwise they become either passive and chair–bound or aggressive through their frustrations. Ideas for coping:

1. The body needs exercise. Many sufferers are physically fit and active; for them walking may be just the right thing, but without a companion they may get lost and become a problem to the family and police.

2. The mind needs to be kept as alert as possible. The carer with all his/her work may not find it possible to give enough time to the patient, but sitters in the home and Day Centre staff should regard it as a priority to ensure that the sufferer does not spend a large amount of time in front of the TV set, or just sleeping. For practical ideas see Sections C4 & 5 pages 39-44.

3. Alzheimer sufferers are able to make a spiritual response just as adults and children can. As they are unable to learn new things, there may be problems for those with no 'religious' background, but the following ideas may be possible:

a) Hymn singing, using old hymns and tunes. Even people who might once have described themselves as 'not religious' may enjoy the hymns that they learnt at school or Sunday School long ago.

b) A simple service can be held at a day centre or residential home using prayers, hymns and readings which are well known. If visitors are invited (local clergy for example) they will need to be primed as to the sort of congregation they will be facing, so that they are not taken aback by unusual responses such as someone wandering around the room.

c) A brief prayer before a visitor leaves.

d) Verses from the Bible or other sacred literature can be

copied out and perhaps done in copperplate or decorated beautifully.

e) Other ideas such as having a communion service for members of a church are more the responsibility of the carer and the clergy, but care attendants and others have a part to play in ensuring that their clients are not forgotten by the church or synagogue just because they don't get out often or behave in an unusual way in the services.

9. MANAGEMENT OF INCONTINENCE

Section B8 dealt with the possible causes of incontinence. Unfortunately a considerable number of Alzheimer sufferers are allowed to suffer incontinence without much attempt to manage the problem. They are being looked after by people who prefer to clear up the shit rather than take steps to prevent the accident in the first place (shortage of staff may be an excuse, but that should not lead to a general policy which has people sitting around in wet or dirty clothes).

The following strategies may prove successful:

a) As part of the care plan for each individual, make sure that he or she goes to the toilet regularly. For some this may mean every two hours during the day; for others every three hours may be more satisfactory. Then it is essential to keep records which can be passed on from shift to shift. Even in the private house this can be done, so that the sitter can take over the system and pass back responsibility to the carer when he/she returns home. Doing this will encourage everybody to think in terms of people being continent, not incontinent.

b) Organise regular movement from one part of the Day Centre/Home to another, and (if possible) pass near the toilet; then ask people if they need to go.

c) Continence pads are available which will keep minor incontinence under control.

d) Some incontinence is, however, caused by slowness of movement. So, to save a few vital seconds, it may help to avoid using buttons and braces and replace them with velcro and elastic – track suit trousers may provide the best answer, even if they are not normally first choice for the elderly.

10. LIFTING

Some sufferers have no difficulty with walking and general mobility, but others may need help to get up out of a chair or to go to the toilet. Some may occasionally fall. Care attendants, home helps and carers too should be taught how to lift without risk to themselves. A local physiotherapist can be asked to give a training session to cover the skills needed for people working on their own or in pairs.

No one on their own should he expected to lift someone from the floor unless the patient is co–operative and able to give a lot of help. Anyone who is a deadweight should be left in a safe and comfortable position while help is got.

There may be a neighbour who is fit enough to assist; if not, you should ring for an ambulance or the police. Unless you feel that the person you are looking after has been injured in the fall you should indicate that it's not an emergency call, but just a pick up.

11. EMERGENCY PROCEDURE FOR CARE ATTENDANTS IN THE HOME (OF USE FOR OTHERS TOO).

In the unlikely event of a sufferer collapsing:

1. Check breathing – resuscitate if breathing has stopped.

2. Stop bleeding at the point of injury (unless there is glass in the wound).

3. Place in the recovery position – unless you suspect that there is a spinal injury or some major fracture.

4. Ensure that the head is to one side and facing downwards so that blood and vomit are not inhaled.

5. Dial 999 – ask for the ambulance service.

6. Report the incident to the carer and your supervisor.

First aid for less serious incidents

1. Know where the first aid kit is kept. If in doubt take one with you.

2. Get advice from your supervisor if you think that a wound or other injury needs to be attended to in casualty. Remember that such a visit will be very confusing for the patient. Using your own car for transporting a patient to hospital may be unwise unless you can find someone to come with you. If you do decide to leave the house to get treatment, make sure that the carer is kept informed somehow, and does not come back to an empty house.

3. Falls – see section C10 on lifting. Reassure the patient and keep him warm.

4. Scalds from kettles etc. should be plunged

immediately in cold (or less hot) water, and will probably need no further treatment. The same applies to minor bruises (e.g. from trapping a finger in a door.)

5. Medicine. No Alzheimer sufferer can be expected to remember to take pills at the right time. So, the sitter must ensure that this is done according to instructions. The carer should be informed that you have done so on his/her return.

12 ALZHEIMER'S PATIENTS LIVING ON THEIR OWN

A lot of elderly people live alone, and considerable numbers suffer from varying degrees of dementia. Without supervision some can be a very great danger to themselves and to others – gas taps, matches, candles, electric fires, paraffin heaters all pose immense problems to Social Workers, Community Psychiatric Nurses, and Home Helps, etc., who may be very aware of potential problems, but may not have any way of ensuring that accidents do not happen.

The Day Centre can be a great help. Staff can ensure that the person eats at least one good meal that day (a lot of sufferers have forgotten how to cook, and don't eat the Meals on Wheels because it comes in a very different way from meals they have eaten in the past), and the stimulation provided by activities and other people, can help to slow down the decline in a person's skills and abilities. Transport may prove to be a problem, as the client may not be ready at the right time, or may not even realise that he/she should be going to the Day Centre on that day at all.

It is open to question whether a sitter service is a proper use of staff if the client is alone. The responsibility element is very much greater when there is no carer to hand over to at the end of the session; it also begs the question of the purpose of the sitter service which is to relieve the carer for a few hours, and not to provide a support which is the responsibility of professionals and the community at large.

The Home Help, however, may be highly involved in the care of such sufferers and have far greater insight into the situation than any other professional or family member. Some Alzheimer patients are perfectly able to function on their own with support, but the Home Help may well become aware of problems which should be mentioned to the Home Help Organiser e.g. signs of incontinence, food hidden away uneaten, misuse of matches etc.

13 ADVOCACY

People with dementia may find it impossible to stand up for themselves. After all they may have very few words that they can use. So when it's a question of a move to a new residential home, they may be quite unable to give their opinions on the matter. For many there will be families or friends who can speak up on their behalf, though some of those relatives and friends may not have their well–being in mind. Others may have nobody in the district who bothers about them; and still others may have nobody in the world. So, for some people there's a need of an advocate, somebody who will speak up loudly to protect the interests of those who have no voice at all.

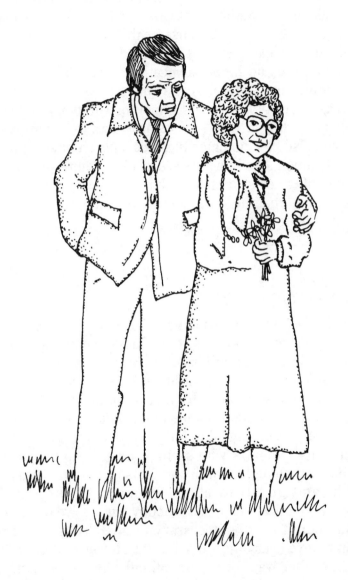

The need seems to be increasing; partly because of the increase in the numbers of people with various forms of dementia; and partly because of the closing of long–stay beds in the Health Service.

And who could be an advocate? Perhaps it's a role for the voluntary sector? Age Concern, the Alzheimer's Disease Society, the local Council of Voluntary Services, as long as they are not service providers themselves. But it could also be a nominee of a local church or synagogue, a trade union, or a business association. There would have to be safeguards to ensure that they were reliable and honest, and that there was some element of supervision of their activities.

14 USE OF DRUGS

There is no cure for Alzheimer's Disease at present. Drug companies are working hard on finding something that is effective in preventing loss of brain function, but there is no magic cure yet. So, the main reason for prescribing drugs is to modify the behaviour of the person. After all a carer who looks after someone on their own all day and every day needs a good night's sleep. And there are some Alzheimer sufferers who seem to manage to keep active all day and all night – or in some cases they stay awake all night and go off to sleep for much of the day. To encourage good sleep, or to modify aggressive or difficult behaviour, it may be necessary to give drugs which will help to give everyone a quieter life. However, there are in theory other ways of coping. Stimulating the person with a range of activities may be an answer; also it may be far better to tire the person out with a long walk so that they develop more normal sleep patterns.

Nursing and rest homes should be in a better position to stimulate their clients both mentally and physically. After all, the staff go home at the end of the shift, and can have a good night's sleep. But a range of activities depends on a generous staffing ratio, and many establishments are unable or unwilling to afford the cost. Their clients are left too much to their own devices, can be difficult, and as a result are kept quiet with drugs. Fortunately there are other homes which go out of their way to make sure that their residents are taken out on visits, and are encouraged to keep as active as possible. I would guess that the amount of drugs used in such places is much lower than in those which make little attempt to stimulate their clients.

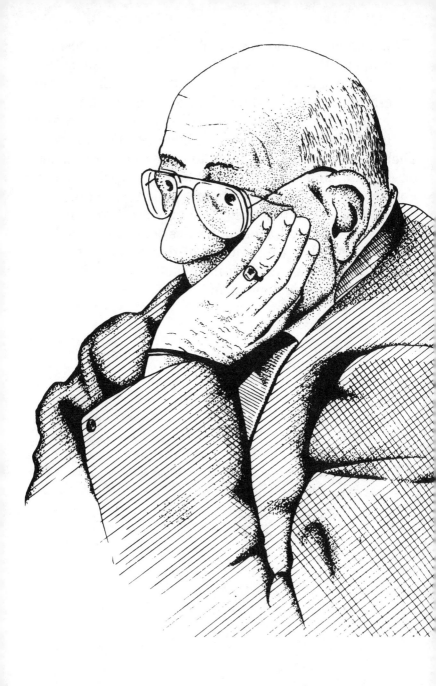

SECTION D

CARERS' PROBLEMS

1. SENSE OF LOSS.

A LIVING BEREAVEMENT

The person you loved has gone. There is no one left to talk to, there is no companionship any more, but at the same time there is a highly demanding person who needs to be fed and dressed and cleaned up. This same loved–one has become (in some cases) unreasonable and cantankerous and unable even to say thank you. At times he doesn't recognise members of his own family and orders them about as if they were servants. His wife is a stranger, whilst there are moments when he mistakes his daughter for his wife.

For some carers there comes the point where they feel that they have been bereaved. The body may require attention, but the real person has departed. Now there may be a permanent feeling of bereavement; the tears may flow,but the period of grieving may be long and drawn–out. The funeral service may be many months or years away, and when death eventually comes, there may be no more tears to shed.

2. TIREDNESS

All work and no play makes Jack a dull boy (and Jill a dull girl). What chance then for Jenny who has a husband and two children, a dog and a hamster to look after as well as her own mother? She would love to get a job now that the children are both at school, but that's out of the question now that her mother demands so much attention. In fact she's got a job, but it's full–time with no breaks, and no pay either. It might be different when the Attendance Allowance comes through for mother; then she'll be able to get the Invalid Care Allowance, which will go some way to help with the family finances, but it isn't what Jenny was looking for; after several years with little children she was looking forward to getting out and about and meeting people. Now she sees even fewer than before.

For Jenny every day is the same – one round of toil from morning to night; but even the night, short as it is, is not reserved for sleep. Granny tends to get up and wander about; she seems to need less and less sleep, and Jenny is the one member of the family who can't sleep through her activity. Anyway, you never know what she's going to do next. So, as Jenny proceeds through towards middle age she finds herself squeezed between her responsibilities as a daughter, mother and wife, and has no time or energy for any activity of her own.

3. LOSS OF CONFIDENCE.

Even highly competent people say that they have felt a massive loss of confidence when they have become carers. Few people know their way round the system; few have the information that they need; few feel confident when faced with experts, even if they are encouraged to be co–workers.

There will come the moment when the carer feels powerless to cope with decisions, or a lack of money, or a feeling of being imprisoned or being put down by someone in authority, or bulldozed by the changes that the planners have brought about in order to give better value for money.

And surprisingly enough, this applies just as much to people in the caring professions as to those who have no idea what a Social Worker does.

But all is not lost. Carers can be very resilient people. And there is many a health worker who has come across the carer who has read up the literature on the illness and has the day–by–day experience to go along with it. Others take a leading part in the activities of the Alzheimer's Disease Society or Age Concern or similar Voluntary organisations.

4. ISOLATION

Most carers become isolated and lonely. Many are themselves in need of care for their own illnesses, and the caring task may put them under increasing pressure until their health breaks.

A pattern of caring for 24 hours a day means that even a short trip to the shops becomes a luxury. Other social activities may gradually become a thing of the past, as the carer goes through a variety of stages which may include embarrassment when the sufferer accompanies them or fear of some disaster if the sufferer stays at home. There are similar feelings about having visitors in the house. While young children may be very understanding, teenagers are likely to be horrified if their friends come to the house while the patient is behaving oddly, and will choose to see them elsewhere. As a result the carer is likely to become even more isolated.

In some ways the carer becomes a sort of non–person, unable to take a proper part in the life of the community around them; forgotten by friends and often family as well; ignored by the busy professional, until they lose confidence in themselves and their abilities.

For the lonely carer, bereavement does not necessarily bring any relief. It may prove very hard indeed to re-enter the world around on your own; it may be impossible to get a job again, and the trip to the DSS to sign on may appear to be a particularly cruel sequel to a career in caring. There is not much chance of adjustment when the allowances disappear overnight and the bills still keep coming in.

5. FAMILY DISUNITY

Mary was very worried about her mother and went across town every day to see her; as Alzheimer's Disease progressed, she found it more and more difficult to get away and tended to arrive home after Richard, her husband, got back from work. He gradually got more and more unsympathetic and threatened to leave her if she carried on spending so much time away from the house. 'Put the old lady in a home' he said. But Mary felt she couldn't do that.

Fred was the only one of the family who hadn't got married; so it seemed natural that he should have Dad to stay with him for a while when he was a bit confused. Fred had just retired, as well, so he hadn't any responsibilities. Soon he found he couldn't get out so easily, and had to get back quickly from the darts match at the Rose & Crown on a Monday night. One Monday he got back a little late and found his sister and her husband George at the house. George was furious, as the old man had gone round to their house in a confused state and knocked them up, when they were getting ready for an early night. 'Don't you leave the old man on his own again, do you hear?' was George's parting shot.

Just two possible scenes from family life, but repeated in a variety of different ways. Apart from the minority who have no wish to be involved with anybody else's problems, why do people behave in such an unhelpful way? No one answer probably, but lack of knowledge and understanding of the sufferer's situation may lie at the root of it. A few suggestions:

1. Get everyone involved to read the Carer's Manual published by the Alzheimer's Disease Society. It is available from them at 10 Greencoat Place London SW1P IPH.

2. Encourage all the family to manage the environment i.e. organise the life of the house as far as possible in a quiet atmosphere around the needs of the patient.

3. Try to get the family to realise that symptoms of Alzheimer's Disease (like wandering and aggression) are not being done on purpose to annoy; it's as much a feature of the illness as a high temperature is a symptom of influenza.

6. ROLE REVERSAL

Parents accept as normal that babies need to be fed and have their nappy changed. These same children when grown–up, may find it nearly impossible to accept the need to feed and clean up their dependent mother or father. It's bad enough to accept that Mum or Dad will never be able to live independently, never be able to write a letter or redecorate a room; it might be difficult helping them to get out of bed or walk down the corridor, but to deal with the most personal of tasks is a reversal of roles that most people don't cope with too easily. A son may never have seen his mother with no clothes on, a daughter may never have expected to have to clean her father up after he'd dirtied the bed, his pyjamas and himself. It may be difficult enough for those who work in nursing homes and hospitals, but at least they are working with someone else's parents, not their own. Somehow it touches the most sensitive area of our inhibitions, and may cause such revulsion that the carer is driven to despair.

And the result? It's easy then to think that the unsocial behaviour is a deliberate attempt to gain attention. The result may be another form of role reversal when the parent gets told off or even punished for 'naughty' behaviour.

The grown-up child needs to accept that there has indeed been a change in role, but to avoid adopting the complete reversal of taking on a parent role; perhaps it should be the 'nurse' or 'care assistant' role which needs to be aimed for, specially at moments of intimate care, changing back to a more mature adult child role which makes it more possible for everyone to be treated with dignity.

7. THE HUSBAND/WIFE RELATIONSHIP

And what about children? When Edward was 15 and growing up through adolescence, his father Nick was 55 and growing downwards through dementia. As they passed each other on this sort of maturity escalator, what emotions did they experience? What sort of a model of manhood and fatherhood did Edward get in those important years as Nick's skills vanished one by one? How do you think he felt when he came home one hot day to find his father sitting in the garden wearing only a hat? How do you think he felt the day when his Dad pushed him aside and rushed through the front door out into the busy street?

Generally speaking, teenagers are not good at dealing with this sort of situation: after all, they have their own growth and behaviour problems to sort out; parents are enough of an embarrassment at the best of times without the added difficulties of a wandering father, or one who could be relied on to say or do the wrong thing.

Little children may find it easier; perhaps they can identify more easily with a Grandmother who is incontinent when they are still having a few accidents. Perhaps they can understand how difficult it is for Grandad to dress himself properly when they get tangled up a bit from time to time. And they may be more patient with him when he gets lost for words as they may have a struggle to say what they want.

8.   ELDER ABUSE

Four in the morning and Auntie May was calling yet again. Mark and Anne had hardly had any sleep at all that night; the old lady had been late to bed, and had woken them up already twice. Soon it would be time for the alarm clock to ring, as Mark was on early turn. This time the bed was soaked and needed to be changed, just like the night before. Anne could stand it no longer. As Auntie May started up again with her nonsense language, she hit her across the face. She knew she should never have done such a thing even before the screams came, and her husband came running, and the children woke up in the room next door. She felt so guilty about the way she had behaved, and tried to make up for it the next day.

Alzheimer's memories may be vanishing, but carers' memories don't go away, and Anne, like many other carers was unable to erase this incident from her mind. But guilty memories don't stop abuse like that happening again. In fact there is a sort of merry–go–round of feelings and behaviour which can go on and on. It starts with a cocktail of anger, fatigue and isolation; then some word or situation triggers abuse of some sort; this is followed by guilty feelings to add to the cocktail. A few days or weeks and something is quite likely to start the cycle off all over again.

In the end abuse may come to light. A hospital admittance, questions asked by the doctor, a chance visit by someone at the wrong moment. What should be done about it? It's easy to think of taking the victim away in order to put an end to the problem. But Auntie May could prefer the security of Anne's loving care to the unknown safe world of a bed in a hospital or nursing home. In fact it can be seen as another form of abuse for her to be taken away at all. What she wants is for the abuse to stop. What Anne needs is a good night's sleep. What community care should be able to offer is enough help to make it possible for Anne to carry on caring without having the cocktail of feelings which she was living with long before the guilt appeared.

And what about abuse by professionals? There is a constant need for standards of care in both public and private sectors to be monitored by management and realistically inspected by Health or Social Services. I do not feel that it is good enough to accept the 'input/output' model of care which is often regarded as good enough practice. I mean by that: ensuring that clients are fed and cleaned up. kept warm and safe. Pressure from outside may encourage the occasional activities session or a quick trip in a mini–bus but otherwise days can be spent just sitting in the lounge or worse still in solitary confinement in the client's bedroom.

That may not seem to be what abuse is about. But lack of stimulation makes the downhill pattern of dementia go even faster and is no less abusive than keeping a young child away from toys and activity.

More obvious abuse may be the result of the desperation of busy staff and management to cope with the many demands of a busy life. Shortage of staff may easily lead to shortness of temper. A slap on the wrist can lead to more forceful methods of control with bruises to show. At its worst there is physical restraint such as tying of people to chairs. It can be justified in the best interests of the client, a sort of safe keeping which can easily become safe custody. That may be a good excuse but it's not a good enough reason for policies which have been used in the past and have yet to disappear totally. What is needed is the imagination and the will to provide a programme of care which suits each individual and which is seen as so important as to require money and time to be spent on it.

Problems don't go away with good practice but they are certainly reduced. If people are looked after as individuals who matter, then there will be less likelihood that they will explode with anger or try to walk off down the road in order to escape.

9. ANGER AND GUILT

When Auntie Ethel asked what time lunch was *she* didn't know she'd asked eight times already. Her niece, Susan, knew because she'd got to the point of counting all

Auntie's questions.

She'd told her eight times that it would be at one o'clock but the ninth time she just lost her cool and told her just where to go. Immediately she wished she'd bitten her tongue, as the old lady burst into tears. How could she have been so unkind? Auntie just forgot each time, and she only wanted to get the answer to a simple question.

George always followed someone around the house and garden. His son Fred usually didn't mind, but one Saturday he wanted to do some work on the car, and every time he turned round, there was Dad just behind him wanting to know what he was doing. After an hour of being patient, Fred got more and more agitated and just pushed his father away – not gently enough though. The old man fell and struck his head on the car as he went down. They asked a lot of questions at Casualty, but Fred managed to persuade them, though for many a night he lay awake and re–lived the events of that dreadful Saturday morning.

Two simple stories of anger and guilt – a natural result of the stress that many carers experience when the frustrations and loneliness and tiredness lead to frayed tempers, and a quick push or a slap or words which are regretted straightaway. For some it can become a way of life, and the old person is battered day after day.

Guilt doesn't only surface when there has been an explosion of anger or an incident which carers can live to regret. There are plenty of other ways in which they can end up having sleepless nights. Henry went out to the Works Dance and left Rosemary behind being looked after by the Crossroads Care Attendant. He enjoyed the company and danced the evening away but when he got home he felt guilty that he should have gone out and enjoyed himself while his dancing partner of the past was left at home.

Katie had never seen her grandchildren who lived in Italy. She longed to get out to Milan to see them; she even started going to Italian classes when her mother was at the Day Centre. So eventually she arranged for a respite care bed in a Nursing Home and was off to the airport for a fortnight with the family and a spot of southern sun. But it was a different story when she got back. Mother was in no state to go back home; she had gone downhill from the very first day and didn't even recognise her own daughter any longer. The funeral was held a month later. 'If only' said Katie 'if only I'd stayed in England, this would never have happened. It's all my fault'. Of course it wasn't all Katie's fault. But that didn't stop her blaming herself for years to come.

10. FINANCE

Being ill is expensive; having an illness like Alzheimer's Disease can seriously damage a carer's wallet. There will be extra fuel bills; furniture and carpets may be damaged; valuable items may disappear (down the loo for example); for those in work, there may be a drop in earning power with a delay while the question of a breakdown pension is investigated. But the biggest problems may come when it is necessary to find full–time care. The situation will I hope change but as I write this in early 1994 it is possible that some carer is being told that the whole of her husband's pension will have to be used in order to finance the place in a Nursing Home that is being arranged. What a reward for her years of caring! What a shock to discover that an income which she regarded as partly hers is being confiscated in order to provide the care that is now beyond her ability. What should she do about it? Too late for the appalling solution shown in the American film 'Do You Remember Love?' where a wife talks about her divorce as the way she had found to avoid financial problems.

11. THE BANK ACCOUNT.

Joe had never refused to sign a cheque. He had not understood for some time what he was doing, but he could always be relied upon to sign his name. But the day came when he had forgotten how to write anything and the cheque for the gas bill remained unsigned. The Bank could not help; the account was only in Joe's name and if he couldn't sign, they were powerless without a Power of Attorney. The lawyer was no help either. No, he couldn't arrange a Power of Attorney without Joe's signature; that wouldn't be possible as Joe had to be able to understand what he was signing. He added that it would have to have been an Enduring Power of Attorney as the ordinary one would be no longer valid now that Joe's dementia was so far advanced. There was now only one thing left to be done. Apply to the Court of Protection for the right to run his affairs. But the Court of Protection does not act in a hurry – for good reasons. Enquiries have to be made and it would take time before that Gas bill (and all the others) could be paid. In the meantime John's wife would have to cope with the problem as best she could.

So it's worth warning carers that they should get the Enduring Power of Attorney as soon as it is clear that their relative is suffering from dementia. Without it they may be in the same position as Joe's wife – quite unable to tap any of the money in the bank account, unable to deal with investments or to sell the house. Not all carers will be in as bad a situation as this. Many will have a joint account; others will have their own savings. But there are bound to be times when both parties are needed to sign a document and without the Enduring Power of Attorney there may well be a long wait for the Court of Protection to come to their aid.

12. DOCTORS AND HOSPITALS

People with Alzheimer's Disease don't go to the doctor. A sweeping statement but generally true. After all they have some insight into their illness at the early stages. They know that their abilities are disappearing and would prefer not to have the doctor tell them the whole truth. So suggestions from carers fall on deaf ears. 'I don't like going to the doctor', 'The doctor can't help with what's wrong with me' – these are just two possible reactions which will avoid the problem for another few weeks. And if the carer is successful in persuading a relative to come to the surgery there is every chance that it will be a wasted journey. For one thing people with dementia are very good at covering up the illness for short periods; they perform particularly well for doctors who are not likely to find anything clinically wrong. After all you don't have a high temperature or raised blood pressure with Alzheimer's Disease. So it may seem as if the carer is just making a fuss – or even that it is the carer who is sick. Of course that may be true; months of looking after someone in the early stages of dementia is a recipe for physical illness for most people. So it would be quite understandable if the 'wrong' patient ended up being treated.

The illness might possibly come to light as a result of

some other medical condition. But if the doctor just sees a 'bronchitis case' or someone suffering from angina the dementia may not be noticed at all or just thought of as a side–effect of a physical illness. (Of course it must be said here that the opposite is also true; there are people who have a physical illness such as a urinary tract infection and behave as if they were suffering from dementia).

It is more likely that the truth will come out as a result of being admitted to an ordinary hospital ward. That may be because of a fall; perhaps a broken leg is the result and the person ends up in a ward along with other fracture cases. Or an operation is needed – perhaps as a result of prostate trouble. And then the difficulties begin.

And there can he difficulties even when it is known that a person is suffering from Alzheimers.

Take John for example. He fell off the toilet and broke his arm. He had been left for several minutes on his own by staff who were probably very busy. Did they know that he was suffering from dementia and that his brain didn't always give the right signals to the muscles; and as a result he often was unable to sit down or stand up? Perhaps not. Perhaps they just saw him as another elderly person brought in for investigations.

Perhaps the ward sister needed to be told that John was probably going to behave in an unusual way because of his dementia and for the staff to be better prepared to deal with him.

But it highlights the special difficulties of looking after people with Alzheimer's Disease in a 'mixed' group of people. In a surgical ward staff are likely to make assumptions about how their patients are going to behave. So to find someone wandering out of the hospital in the middle of the night or trying to get into someone else's bed is not something they are expecting – nor something that their training has prepared them for. It can also be an unpleasant shock for the patient in the next bed to have his meal stolen while he wasn't looking!

It may be all too easy to think that the patient is being difficult on purpose but if staff have been given full information about the dementia then confusion and unusual behaviour should be expected. After all, the change in surroundings can be difficult enough for anybody, but for someone like John it can feel as if he has lost his home and the person who was looking after him as well.

13. THE CARER'S HEALTH

The carer's breakdown in health may also create a crisis. Mary was only due to be away from home for a short while for a minor operation, plus a few days to get over it. It seemed a good idea for James, her husband to go to a local Nursing home while she couldn't look after him. But James didn't understand why he was in a strange unfamiliar home nor why his beloved Mary wasn't around any longer. By the time that Mary was fit enough to take up her duties as chief carer again James had gone downhill so much that there was no way that he would be able to cope in the house. So James stayed in his Nursing Home; and Mary? With no James to look after she suffered a breakdown herself and claimed that 'they' had kidnapped her husband; she was admitted to the Psychiatric ward where she quickly died after refusing all food and drink. Over five or six years James had been the centre of her life; she had been nurse and care attendant housekeeper and chauffeur. Her operation had taken all this away from her; so she blamed herself for the situation and then transferred the blame on to 'them'.

Probably nothing would have prevented Mary's crisis; she received all the support that could be expected while she was looking after James; however there are plenty of other carers who spend years caring for someone with little help from anybody. They may find that they are hardly noticed by the professionals they open the door to; this seems to be specially true for women who may just feel taken for granted. Their health may be vastly improved if they realise that the doctor, the nurse and the social worker all have their well-being in mind when they come to visit, as well as the well-being of their relative. It might be even better if they were regarded as the key worker who should be consulted and included in discussions.

Ignore the carer and you may have two people needing emergency help; for if the carer goes into hospital the person being cared for will also need a bed somewhere and there may be no going back when the carer has recovered.

14. CARE OF THE CARER

Some suggestions for helping carers cope.

1. Make sure that they are getting as much support as possible from friends neighbours and family, who need to be kept informed of the problems they are experiencing.

2. Make sure they are getting as much help as possible from Social and Health Services and also voluntary organisations such as the Alzheimer's Disease Society and Crossroads.

3. They might find it a good use of the Invalid Care

Allowance to pay for someone to come in and sit with their relative on a regular basis.

4. The carer needs regular breaks and holidays. Some areas provide respite care in one or more of the following patterns:

   a) Admission to a holiday bed in a hospital.

   b) A bed in a Home for the Elderly run by the Local Authority.

   c) A bed in a specialist nursing home paid for by the Health Authority.

   d) A fostering scheme whereby the sufferer goes to a family who lives nearby who provide care in an ordinary home. This is best done on a regular and frequent basis such as every three weeks.

   e) Both carer and sufferer go away together to a hotel or guest house which is designed and prepared for the problems which may arise. The best way of finding out what is available is from: Holiday Care Service, 2 Old Bank Chambers, Station Road, Horley, Surrey RH6 9HW. Tel: 01293 774535. Please enclose a stamped addressed envelope.

   f) The ideal is care in the person's own home provided by either a member of the family or by someone who is prepared to undertake a 24 hour a day job for a week or so.

Unfortunately the move from home to hospital or other form of institutional care tends to be a very confusing episode for someone suffering from Alzheimer's Disease, and many go quickly downhill, a situation which causes many carers to feel even more guilty that they should have abandoned their loved one and actually enjoyed themselves for a few days.

If your job takes you into the home, you may be the only person a carer may see for more than a minute or two. His/her main need may be to spend time talking, and so a major job for the home help, care attendant etc. may be to sit and listen. Other professionals may always appear to be in a hurry, but you can afford to spend time.

However, if the carer comes back after shopping and does not appreciate that the sitter has a family to return to, or another carer to go to, it may be advisable to make up a programme which suits the situation. For example:

Day 1   Preliminary visit.

Day 2   Arrange a handing-over period when you arrive. The carer goes out for about $1^1/_2$ hours, followed by 20 minutes for a chat over a cup of tea.

Day 3   Shorten the final chat time.

Day 4   5 minutes hand-over at the beginning.

$1 \, ^3/_4$ hours carer out.

10 minutes to talk on his/her return

The carer may be in need of information which care attendants can be in a good position to give; some can be found in this book or the Alzheimer's Disease Society manual. Advice is more difficult and dangerous too, especially if it turns out to be bad advice. It should always be the carer who makes up his/her mind about major decisions; the job of all the professionals who talk with the carer is to make all the various issues clearer, not to impose decisions on other people.

15. A CARER CARD

When the staff at the supermarket came to lock up the car park at night they found a car in one of the bays. Inside was an elderly lady, very agitated and confused. She had clearly been there some time; she mentioned a name – Henry. Suddenly it dawned on one of the supermarket staff. It was a 'Henry' who had been taken to hospital after collapsing at the check–out – and that was in mid–afternoon. So for several hours Henry's wife had sat in the car waiting for her husband who by closing time was being pronounced dead of a heart attack.

Carers often worry that they will be taken ill or have an accident while they are out; and naturally they are afraid that the person they look after will be left alone for a long time.

One solution is a numbered card which says: My wife suffers from dementia; if I am taken ill or have an accident please contact....... This is followed by the name and phone number of a Residential Home which has agreed to run the service. The Home would have the list of names matching the numbers on the cards, and they would be in a position to alert others to the fact that someone with Alzheimer's Disease was on their own, perhaps at home, perhaps like Henry's wife in a car in a deserted car park.

16. LIFELINE

Carers may worry about an accident when they are out. They ought to be equally worried about the same thing happening when they are in the safety of their own homes. Lifeline (and other similar systems) may be seen as intended for people who live on their own, a way of attracting attention in cases of emergency. But if you look after someone with Alzheimer's Disease, then you ARE on your own; nobody else will dial 999; nobody else will run next door for help. so, it would be wise to have some way of calling for assistance, like an alarm button on a pendant which can be worn in the house and garden.

For further information contact your local Housing Department who may well run a local service. Or nationally there is the Tunstall Alarm System.

17. GIVING UP

Carers often give up – they give up going to see friends, going to the pub or to church; they stop playing golf and bowls; they rarely entertain; they resign from membership of committees and sometimes their jobs as well.

But they find it very difficult to give up caring for a relative or friend. As the world closes in around them they generally manage to find the strength and energy to carry on.

But the day eventually comes when full–time care becomes necessary Sometimes this comes about as a result of an accident or illness. It becomes clear even to the carer that they can't continue the round–the–clock caring in circumstances that require two people to carry out the work. But often it is a more gradual process, which can be planned for. It might be helpful to have a round–table conference with one or two other members of the family, Social Worker, Care Assistant, Doctor, District Nurse etc, who could help to come to a decision as to the best way forward.

Support continues to be needed when the carer finally says goodbye. It's a further sort of bereavement which will not be helped if all the professionals stop visiting immediately. One thing that will be needed in some cases is help with transport to get to the hospital or nursing home. For most carers are regular visitors (sometimes even when it's a respite care admission) and may set themselves the target of visiting on a daily basis whatever the weather. But they will also need emotional support to be able to cope with the empty chair in the corner.

And whose fault is it that the chair is empty? It's quite possible that they will think that they should take the blame because their relative would still be there, if they had been able to carry on caring.

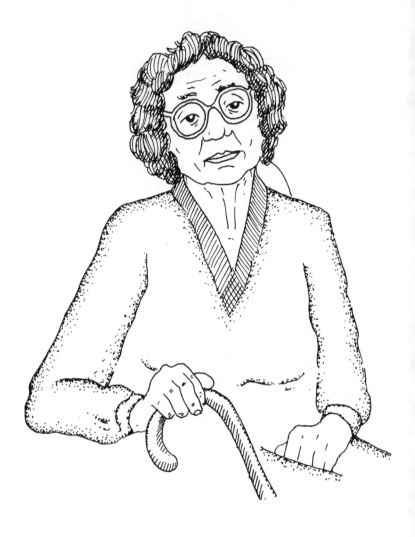

SECTION E

THE SUPPORT SERVICES

1. HEALTH

a) Family Doctor – General Practitioner – G.P. The gatekeeper to most of the services in the Health Service and a way of being referred to the Social Services. He/she should refer possible dementia sufferers to a psycho–geriatrician for diagnosis. If Alzheimer's Disease is diagnosed the GP should make every effort to see that the carer is supported in his/her caring job, otherwise there will be two patients to be cared for instead of one.

b) The District Nurse can be called in by the GP to deal with dressings, incontinence pads, bathing etc. The Health Visitor can also be involved in giving advice on health care (though her case load is made up mainly of children under 5).

c) The Geriatrician is an expert in the care of the elderly. He sometimes has to deal with the confused elderly if there is no specialist Psycho–geriatrician in the area. The Psycho–geriatrician looks after dementia patients who are over 65 and in some areas takes on all cases of Alzheimer's Disease regardless of age. But in other areas the under 65 Alzheimer patient becomes the responsibility of the Psychiatrist.

d) The Community Psychiatric Nurse works closely with the Psycho–geriatrician, as does the Medical Social Worker.

e) The Physiotherapist's skills provide exercises which keep the muscles in good shape.

f) The Occupational Therapist can advise on equipment and adaptations in the home and help clients to retain their everyday skills and interests for as long as possible.

g) The Psychologist deals with the workings of the mind. He also will run Reality Orientation sessions which will aim to ensure that sufferers are made aware of the real world about them and are not left in a total fantasy world. The psychologist may also run a Relatives' Support Group to enable people to share their problems and experiences. Equally staff may need to have a psychologist's help with talking through the problems which they have in the stress and strain of dealing with difficult and demanding patients.

h) The Continence Service is a rarity, but it's worth asking about it. There may be one available in your area.

2. DSS – DEPARTMENT OF SOCIAL SECURITY.

This is NOT the place to go to talk to a Social Worker or get a Home Help. It deals with benefits such as:

> Disability Living Allowance
> Invalid Care Allowance
> Attendance Allowance
> Help towards Nursing Home fees
> and loans from the Social Fund.

3. SOCIAL SERVICES

The Social Worker is employed by the Local Authority, and is often based at a local (or patch) office. At the main office there is a duty Social Worker who attends to calls during normal working hours. Everyone has a right to a Social Worker without being referred by someone else.

The Social Worker is a gatekeeper to services such as a Home Help, Laundry Service, Homes for the Elderly, Day Centres, Meals on Wheels.

Day Centres are often organised by the Social Services who are able to make use of part of a Home for the Elderly for this purpose; they may also be run by voluntary bodies like the Alzheimer's Disease Society. Day Hospitals are run by the Health Authority and are intended to be used for assessing confused people without removing them totally from their home.

Sitter service – the main agency in the country which offers a sitter or befriending service is Crossroads which has more than a hundred branches in the United Kingdom; their's is a service available to people with a wide range of disabilities. In some areas the Alzheimer's Disease Society offers a specialist service with staff specifically trained in the needs of people with Alzheimer's. There are also a number of private organisations which offer a similar service.

All staff should be trained before they take on their first visit.

The purpose of a sitter service is twofold:

a) to let the carer go out and do some shopping or have a meal in a restaurant or go to the cinema (or alternatively stay at home and get on with a hobby or re-decorate a room or do some gardening without having to worry about their dependant).

b) to look after the sufferer, encourage conversation and

activity. It does not involve housework apart from the preparation of a snack or an activity like cooking which is beneficial to the sufferer.

Local Authority Home for the Elderly –
Some areas have specialist homes for the confused elderly; others have a policy of putting a small group of confused people in each home.

4. HOMES FOR THE ELDERLY

Until recently these were mainly run by Social Services departments; but now the private sector is expanding, though the provision is very uneven in the country, with large numbers of homes in some seaside towns, but very few in large urban areas. In some cases there are specialist homes for people suffering from dementia. They may be given a range of different titles: EMI (Elderly Mentally Infirm); EMF (Elderly Mentally Frail); the confused elderly.

In other cases there is a policy of mixing different sorts of people, with people with dementia in the same establishment and the same sitting room as people with other sorts of disability and need.

There are also long-stay beds available in some hospitals for the elderly or in the few remaining mental hospitals.

In the private sector there are two sorts of care on offer. The Rest Home which offers very little nursing care; the Nursing Home which may take very dependent people and which has to have a qualified nurse on duty at all times. Some Rest Homes and Nursing Homes specialise in dementia, but others may refuse to keep someone with difficult or aggressive behaviour; they feel that they do not have the resources to cope adequately, and may be worried about the effects on other residents. Lists of Rest and Nursing Homes can be obtained from Social Services or from a Medical Social Worker at a hospital.

The local authority is responsible for the registration and inspection of Rest Homes; and the Health Authority is responsible for registration and inspection of Nursing Homes.

5. VOLUNTARY ORGANISATIONS.

The Alzheimer's Disease Society is the specialist society dealing with all types of dementia (apart from Huntington's Chorea for which there is a separate society). It has a London headquarters and branches in many part of the country, some of which run Day Centres and sitter services. Members receive a monthly newsletter to help them keep in touch with developments in research and in services for dementia sufferers and their carers.

Scotland has its own organisation entitled 'Alzheimer's Scotland' with a headquarters in Edinburgh.

There is also an Alzheimer's International based in America; every year there is a conference hosted by a different country. There are Alzheimer Societies in most of the larger European countries and also in Australia, New Zealand, Canada, America, Singapore, Japan and India.

For some addresses please see page 92.

Carers' National Association: this is the single voice of carers throughout the country. It has a London headquarters with a number of branches.

Crossroads care is based in Rugby. It provides for Care staff to visit homes to do tasks ranging from getting people up in the morning to sitting with someone while their carer has a few hours break. They do not specialise in Alzheimer's Disease, but will include many Alzheimer's families among their clients.

Council of Voluntary Service. Most areas have an umbrella organisation which promotes voluntary groups of all sorts. They may have information about local activities of organisations which may be actively supporting people with Alzheimer's Disease. These might include the following; Mind, Age Concern, Help the Aged.

Churches. Most large denominations have a social responsibility department either centrally organised or in each region. The local situation will probably be very mixed, but it's often useful to contact the priest or minister who may be able to ask some suitable volunteer to assist.

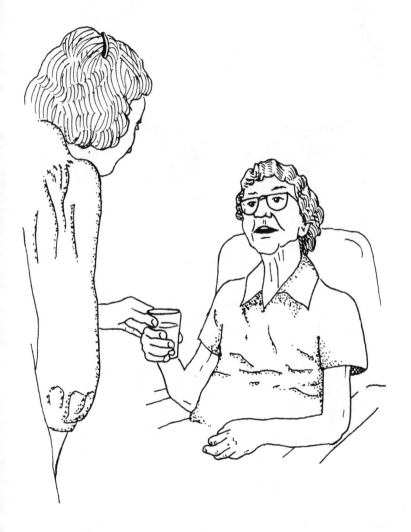

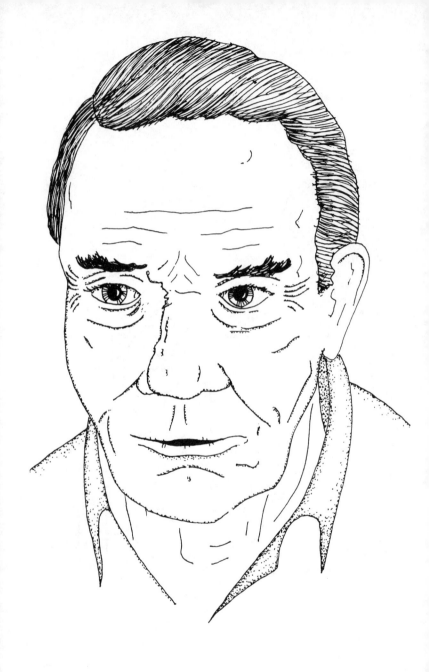

SECTION F

POSSIBLE CAUSES OF ALZHEIMER'S DISEASE

For those who visit carers in their homes the question of the cause of the illness will sooner or later come up. This is partly because carers sometimes feel that they have been responsible for the condition of their loved one.

For example, problems may begin to be obvious soon after retirement and a move to a new house. The partner begins to ask whether the change in lifestyle can be blamed for the situation; and, also, whether they can blame themselves for the decision to retire and move, or whether some other action of theirs has triggered off the illness.

Unfortunately, at present there is no clear answer. However, there are a number of theories, all of which might turn out to be valid, for Alzheimer's Disease is quite likely to have more than one single cause.

So, here are five theories:

1. The family factor. There are families which seem to have a large number of people with Alzheimer's Disease down the generations. But most sufferers do not come from such families. And, the families which are affected also have members who miss getting the disease.

2. People with Alzheimer's Disease have traces of aluminium in their brain. In fact these are described as aluminium plaques. How did they get there? Was it alu-

minium in the water supply? There is aluminium naturally in water in many parts of the country, and it is sometimes added as well. So, perhaps it has something to do with what we eat and drink. However, aluminium can also be found in the brains of people who have not shown signs of dementia.

3. A long time virus; that is, one that takes many years rather than days to incubate. There are some rare dementias like this, but we don't know if this is a cause in Alzheimer's Disease.

4. An environmental factor? Nobody knows, but it's always possible.

5. A major life event? Perhaps the disease could be triggered off by something like the loss of a job, or maybe an accident, or an operation. Was it caused by retirement or the death of a close friend or relative? Or was the illness revealed when lifestyle changed in the days following the event?

6. Is it a combination of several causes? Maybe a family factor which needs something else to cause the illness to make its appearance.

To obtain reliable information about the latest medical research, it pays to be a member of the Alzheimer's Disease Society. Membership includes the monthly newsletter which features regular articles about medical research into the illness.

ALZHEIMER'S DISEASE AND OTHER DEMENTIAS

Alzheimer's Disease covers the majority of cases of dementia. Until a few years ago it was thought of as a rare disease among younger people, that is, under the age of 65; there was also a feeling that dementia was more or less normal at some stage in old age. But however much we may lose brain cells as the years go by, it is nothing in comparison with the huge losses in the brain of those who suffer from dementia. And the losses can occur at any age from about 40 onwards; the pattern may be different at 49 and 79 but the effects are likely to be similar.

About 20% of dementia sufferers have a version known as multi–infarct dementia; that is, they have had a series of mini–strokes which seem to have knocked out certain vital functions of the brain. Some of these may not matter at all, but others can lead to dependence on other people. For example a sudden inability to read or write may alter someone's lifestyle considerably. Or incontinence may make it impossible to continue with social life, or even to invite friends back home.

In addition there is a range of other causes – dementia affects a small number of people who have had a stroke; equally some Parkinson's disease sufferers suffer from dementia (or do they just have Alzheimer's as well?). Some of those who have Aids suffer from dementia in the last stages of their illness. Some alcoholics and some boxers may have dementia in later life. And, in addition there are the rare dementias like Pick's Disease and Kreuztfeldt–Jakob syndrome.

DEMENTIA SYMPTOMS WITH OTHER DISEASES

It is possible to think that someone is starting to show the symptoms of dementia, when in fact they are really suffering from something else – maybe an illness which can be cured or controlled. For example:

Elderly people suffering from a urinary infection or bronchitis may be unable to look after themselves properly, may be incontinent and may be difficult to understand. However, they are not suffering from dementia. Proper treatment for their medical condition will clear up their confusion and other symptoms in a few days.

Some people with clinical depression show signs of dementia. If the depression can be kept under control, the dementia symptoms will go away. However, people who are in the early stages of Alzheimer's Disease may have a great awareness of their own failures and may therefore get depressed about the way they are losing their grip.

There are some older people, specially those who look after themselves, who do not eat properly. A poor diet may lead to a loss of some faculties. But, improve the nutrition and the dementia symptoms will disappear. The particular vitamin which is essential to the good order of the brain is B_{12}, which is to be found as a trace element in foods like corn flakes, rise krispies and liver.

Lack of stimulation may give the impression of dementia. Stimulation is good for the brain; it slows down the dementia process and is one reason why people with the illness should be encouraged to keep as active as possible. People who have no brain disease at all may well show some sign of deterioration if they spend all day on their own in their bedroom or are brought down to the lounge of a rest home and left in a chair all day long.

Some symptoms of dementia are caused by a drug cocktail. Elderly people may be prescribed a range of different drugs for a range of conditions and may develop symptoms of dementia as a result. Remove the drugs, and you remove the dementia, but this needs to be done under medical supervision, as some or all of them may be vital.

ADDRESSES

Alzheimer's Disease Society
Gordon House, 10 Greencoat Place, London SW1P 1PH.
Tel: 0171 306 0606

Alzheimer's Scotland
8 Hill Street, Edinburgh EH2 3JZ.
Tel: 0131 225 1453. Helpline 0131 220 6155

Alzheimer International
919 N. Michigan Avenue, Chicago, Illinois, 606011–1676,
USA.
Tel: 312 335 8700

Alzheimer Society of Ireland
St John of God Hospital, Stillorgan, Co Dublin, Ireland.
Tel: 010 353 12 881282

Carers' National Association
20–25 Glasshouse Yard, London EC1A 4JS.
Tel: 0171 490 8818. Carersline 0171 490 8898

Crossroads Care Attendant Scheme
10 Regent Place, Rugby, Warwickshire CV21 2PN.
Tel: 01788 573653

Age Concern
1268 London Road, Nobury, London SW16 4EJ.
Tel: 0181 679 8000

LAST WORD

I have made no mention of a cure for Alzheimer's Disease; and for that I make no apology even if readers may find that they are asked about it by the relatives and friends of those they are caring for. It's not within the scope of this book, neither is it something that I am qualified to write about. Research is gathering pace both in Britain and other countries. A good way of keeping abreast of the situation is to be a member of the Alzheimer's Disease Society, whose monthly Newsletter usually includes an article on some aspect of research. See page 92 for addresses.